# HOME EXERCISES FOR SENIORS OVER 50

Easy-to-follow steps to stay healthy, strong and independent

## PETER ROMAN

# Introduction

Salutations from "SilverFit: Exercise for Seniors Over 50," a book that aims to empower seniors to begin a wellness journey in the convenience of their own homes. Keeping an active lifestyle as we become older is essential to retaining energy and improving general health.

This book offers a curated collection of exercises specifically designed for seniors, focusing on flexibility, strength, and balance. Whether you're a seasoned fitness enthusiast or just beginning your fitness journey, these routines cater to various fitness levels. Embrace the opportunity to enhance your physical well-being, boost energy levels, and foster a positive mindset through simple, effective home exercises. With SilverFit, age becomes a companion to a vibrant and fulfilling life, emphasizing that it's never too late to prioritize your health and well-being.

Let's embark on a journey to enhance your vitality, boost your mood, and foster a sense of well-being through the power of home exercise. Age is just a number, and it's never too late to prioritize your health and enjoy an active fulfilling life.

# Why you need this book

Unlock the Golden Years: A Vital Guide to Home Exercise for Seniors Over 50" is more than just a book; it's your own key to a better, more fulfilled life. In an era where wellness is paramount, this guide stands out as an indispensable companion for those navigating the unique terrain of aging.

Why do you need this book? It's a question of reclaiming control over your health and well-being. Tailored specifically for individuals aged 50 and beyond, this guide addresses the nuanced needs of seniors, offering a diverse array of exercises that prioritize flexibility, strength, and balance. The carefully curated routines are adaptable, ensuring accessibility for various fitness levels – whether you're a fitness enthusiast or just starting your journey.

This book goes beyond the physical aspects of exercise; it delves into the mental and emotional benefits, emphasizing the profound impact on mood, cognitive function, and overall quality of life. As we age, maintaining independence becomes a priority, and these exercises are designed to enhance daily functionality and prevent common age-related issues.

With clear instructions, motivational insights, and a focus on creating joyful exercise habits, "Unlock the Golden Years" becomes your roadmap to an active and fulfilling life. It's a reminder that age is not a limitation but an opportunity to prioritize your health. Invest in yourself, embrace the transformative power of home exercise, and embark on a journey toward a healthier, happier you. This book is your compass, guiding you through the golden years with vitality and purpose.

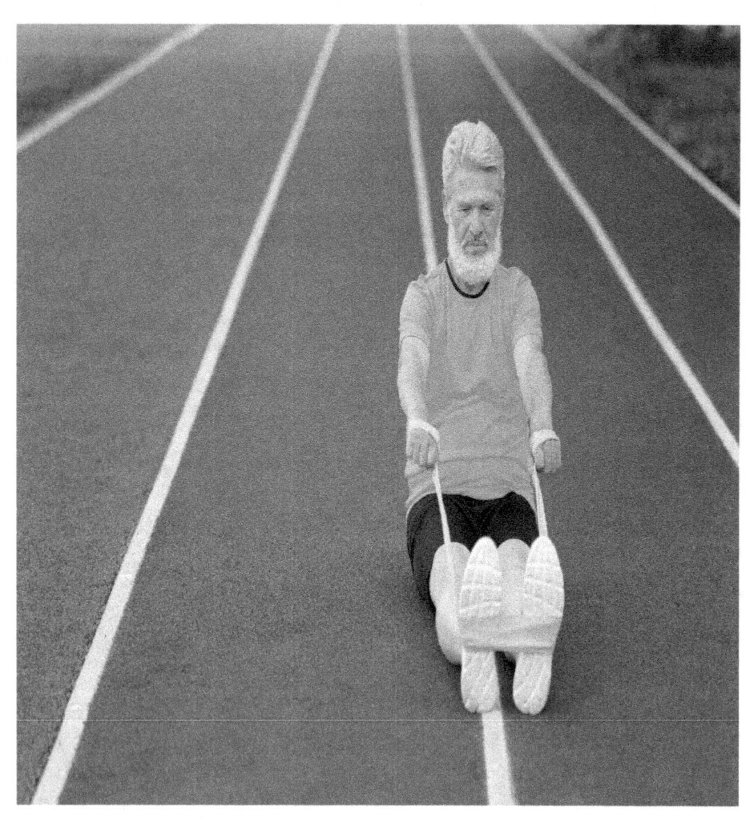

# CHAPTER ONE

## Living the life you want

Home Exercise for Seniors Over 50 encapsulates a holistic approach to fitness and well-being, tailored specifically for individuals navigating the golden years. This philosophy goes beyond mere exercise routines; it's a book designed to empower seniors to lead a life aligned with their desires and optimal health.

Personalized Fitness:
The guide recognizes the diverse needs of seniors aged 50 and above. It provides exercises focused on improving flexibility, strength, and balance, acknowledging that each individual's fitness journey is unique. The emphasis is on personalized routines that cater to various fitness levels.

Comprehensive Well-Being:
This book extends its focus beyond physical health. It acknowledges the interconnected nature of mental, emotional, and physical well-being. The exercises are curated not just to keep the body active but to enhance mood, cognitive function, and overall life satisfaction.

Functional Independence:
A key principle of the book is promoting exercises that enhance daily functionality. By incorporating

movements relevant to daily life, it aims to improve functional independence, contributing to a lifestyle that supports autonomy and minimizes the risk of common age-related challenges.

Joyful Engagement:
Exercise should be a source of joy. This guide encourages seniors to find pleasure in physical activity, whether through activities they love or by exploring new forms of movement. By fostering a positive and enjoyable exercise experience, it aims to establish habits that contribute to long-term well-being.

Beyond Physical Health:
This book  transcends the purely physical aspects of exercise. It delves into mental and emotional well-being, recognizing the profound impact of movement on mood, cognitive function, and overall life satisfaction.

Long-Term Health Focus:
"Living the Life You Want" looks at exercise as a sustainable investment in long-term health. It explores how consistent physical activity contributes to overall well-being, emphasizing the cumulative benefits that lead to a healthier, more fulfilling life in the years to come.

 This book is an invitation for seniors to embrace a lifestyle that prioritizes their unique needs, celebrates their individual journey, and empowers them to live the life they truly desire. It's not just about exercise; it's about fostering a holistic approach to well-being that resonates with the essence of a fulfilling and joyful life.

## How Exercising helps you alive

Regular exercise for seniors over 50 is crucial for maintaining overall health and well-being, especially when done in the comfort of one's home. Engaging in a consistent home exercise routine offers numerous benefits that contribute to a longer and healthier life.

Firstly, regular physical activity helps seniors maintain a healthy weight, reducing the risk of chronic conditions such as heart disease and diabetes. As metabolism tends to slow with age, exercise becomes a powerful tool for managing weight and preserving muscle mass. This is particularly important for seniors as it enhances mobility and reduces strain on joints, promoting a more active lifestyle.

Furthermore, home exercises tailored for seniors focus on improving balance and flexibility, reducing the risk of falls and fractures. Many routines include gentle movements and stretches that enhance joint mobility and overall stability. This is crucial for seniors, as falls can have severe consequences for this age group, often leading to a decline in independence.

Moreover, exercising at home provides a convenient and accessible way for seniors to stay active. It eliminates barriers like transportation issues and weather conditions, making it easier for individuals to adhere to their exercise regimen. This consistency is key to reaping the full benefits of physical activity, from enhanced cardiovascular health to improved mental well-being.
In addition to the physical benefits, home exercises for seniors promote mental health by reducing stress and anxiety. Participating in constant physical activity releases endorphins, which are natural mood enhancers. This is especially important for older adults who may face challenges like isolation or loss of social connections.
incorporating home exercises into the routine of seniors over 50 is a holistic approach to maintaining health. From physical fitness to mental well-being, regular exercise contributes significantly to a vibrant and fulfilling life, allowing seniors to age gracefully and enjoy an active lifestyle within the familiar and comfortable environment of their homes.

# CHAPTER TWO

## Putting in order your body and mind

Carefully assess each senior's specific demands in order to ensure that they participate in at-home exercise. It's critical to modify exercise regimens to account for any current medical concerns, such as arthritis or heart problems. Walking, swimming, light yoga, and some stretching are examples of low-impact exercises that might be great options.
It is important to emphasize strength training, balance, and flexibility. These components support general wellbeing and lessen the risk of falls, which is a major worry for senior citizens. Exercises that increase muscular tone and joint mobility can improve day-to-day functionality.
More important than intensity is consistency. Seniors can safely increase their strength and endurance with gradual improvement. Promoting frequent, shorter sessions as opposed to occasional, long ones helps people stay motivated and avoid burnout.
Exercises should be tailored to each person's tastes and physical capabilities. Personalization is essential. Incorporating pleasurable pursuits like dance or gardening might enhance the routine's engagement. Long-term adherence is also

facilitated by cultivating a positive outlook on exercise.

Safety concerns are crucial, and they include appropriate warm-ups and cool-downs. Consulting with medical experts guarantees that the workouts selected comply with medical guidance. Finally, creating a welcoming atmosphere at home—perhaps with the help of a family member or workout partner—can improve the experience and promote consistency in leading an active lifestyle.

## Preparing smartly

Preparing smartly for home exercises for seniors over 50 involves a thoughtful approach to ensure both safety and effectiveness. First and foremost, a consultation with healthcare professionals is crucial. This ensures that the chosen exercises align with any existing health conditions, medications, or physical limitations.

Creating a dedicated workout space at home enhances focus and safety. This area should be well-lit, clutter-free, and equipped with any necessary supportive tools like handrails or stable chairs for balance exercises. Ensuring proper ventilation and comfortable temperature contributes to a conducive environment.

Selecting exercises that cater to individual needs is paramount. Emphasis should be on a well-rounded routine covering flexibility, balance, and strength training. Low-impact activities, such as seated exercises, yoga, or aquatic exercises, are often well-suited for seniors, reducing the risk of injury. Incorporating suitable warm-ups and cool-downs is essential for preventing strains and enhancing flexibility. Gentle stretches before and after the workout prepare the body and aid in recovery. Monitoring intensity levels is equally important; seniors should gradually progress to avoid overexertion.

Utilizing technology, such as instructional videos designed for seniors, can provide guidance and motivation. Moreover, establishing a consistent schedule helps make exercise a habitual part of daily life. Encouraging social interaction, whether virtually or with a workout partner, adds a supportive and enjoyable aspect to the routine. Seniors should plan ahead for at-home workouts by incorporating these components: health assessment, a dedicated training area, customized exercises, appropriate warm-ups, technological integration, and a regular timetable. This will help them maintain a healthy and productive fitness regimen.

## Using a Simple Exercise Journal

Seniors over 50 who exercise at home may find that keeping a basic exercise journal is helpful. Start by recording the specifics of every training session, such as the exercises done, how long they lasted, and any noteworthy observations. This helps to customize upcoming routines and gives a concrete record of progress.

Provide a space where you can record your body's feelings both before and after each session. This self-evaluation can be used to track improved flexibility and energy levels, pinpoint areas for improvement, or spot possible discomfort. These realizations help create a more individualized and successful fitness program.Tracking consistency is crucial. Use the journal to mark scheduled workout days and note any deviations. This not only instills a sense of accomplishment but also serves as motivation to maintain a regular exercise routine. Record any modifications or adjustments made to the exercises. This information aids in understanding which activities are most comfortable and effective, allowing for ongoing refinement of the workout routine.

Incorporate a brief reflection section where seniors can jot down their overall mood and satisfaction after completing each workout. This emotional component helps foster a positive mindset and reinforces the connection between exercise and well-being.Utilize the journal to set realistic goals and celebrate achievements. Whether it's increasing the duration of a particular exercise or reaching a milestone in strength training, recognizing progress enhances motivation and commitment.

Regularly review the exercise journal, ideally on a weekly or monthly basis. This retrospective analysis aids in identifying trends, adjusting goals, and ensuring the exercise routine continues to align with personal health objectives. Overall, a simple exercise journal serves as a practical and empowering tool for seniors, enhancing the effectiveness and enjoyment of their home exercise regimen.

## Overcoming Home Exercise Barriers

It is imperative that seniors over 50 overcome obstacles to home exercise in order to sustain a regular and beneficial fitness regimen. Motivation is one issue that many people face. To counter this, make sure your exercise routine includes enjoyable activities and that your goals are reasonable and attainable. Making a virtual or in-person connection with a workout partner can increase accountability and add a social and engaging element to the workout.

The absence of a dedicated training area is another obstacle. Establish a distinct space for exercise at home by designating an area, no matter how small. This reduces distractions and aids seniors in mentally getting ready for their workout.

Safety concerns may pose a hurdle. Consult with healthcare professionals to address any medical considerations and ensure exercises align with individual health conditions. Additionally, investing in simple safety equipment, like non-slip mats or stable chairs for support, can enhance the overall safety of the home exercise environment.

One common barrier is time constraints. Seniors can get around this by dividing their exercise regimens into shorter, more doable sessions spaced out throughout the day. This method lowers the chance of fatigue and preserves energy levels while fitting into a busy schedule.

Additionally, boredom can undermine consistency. Exercise routines can be kept interesting and fresh by experimenting with different exercises, adding music or podcasts, and trying new things. Examining online courses or senior-focused instructional videos can also offer diversity and direction.

Addressing physical discomfort is crucial. Gradual progress in intensity and modify exercises as needed to prevent strain or injury. Regular check-ins with healthcare professionals can help tailor the routine to accommodate any changing health considerations.

By acknowledging and addressing these barriers, seniors can create a more supportive and sustainable home exercise routine, enhancing their overall well-being.

# CHAPTER THREE

## Flexibility Exercise

Flexibility exercises are crucial for seniors over 50, promoting joint health, reducing stiffness, and enhancing overall mobility. Performing these exercises at home is convenient and supports a more active lifestyle.

Start with gentle warm-up activities like shoulder circles, neck tilts, and ankle rotations. These movements prepare the body for flexibility exercises, preventing injury.

Dynamic stretches, such as arm swings and leg swings, are beneficial for seniors as they engage various muscle groups and gradually increase range of motion. These can be easily incorporated into a home routine, requiring minimal space.

Static stretches are equally important and involve holding a stretch for a prolonged period. Focus on major muscle groups like hamstrings, quadriceps, and calf muscles. Seniors should perform these stretches within a pain-free range, gradually progressing over time.

Aim for at least 10-15 minutes of flexibility exercises, 2-3 times per week. Regular practice helps maintain and improve flexibility, supporting daily activities and reducing the risk of falls.

# Gentle stretching

Mild stretching improves mobility overall, relieves stiffness, and promotes flexibility. Here's a quick guide to help you add some light stretching to your regimen:

1.Stretches for the neck: Tilt the head gently from side to side, holding each posture for a short while.
   - To relieve tension, slowly turn the neck clockwise and then counterclockwise.

2. Stretching for the Upper Back and Shoulders:
   - Move the shoulders in a circular motion, back and forth.
   - To stretch the shoulders and upper back, bring your hands together in front of you and raise your arms.

3. Arm and Wrist Stretches: - Stretch out one arm in front of you while using the other hand to gently pull your fingers toward your body.
   - Swivel wrists in a clockwise and counterclockwise direction.

4. Spine Stretch: – Take a tall stance or sit, then slowly rotate your torso to one side, holding the pose for a few seconds. Continue on the opposite side.

5. Hip and Thigh Stretches:– To extend the thighs, lift your legs while seated.

- For balance, stand close to a solid object. Raise one knee to the chest and hold it there for a little while.

6. Strolling the Ankles and Calf:
   - To stretch your calf, stand facing a wall, place your hands on it, and take a straight step back.
   - While seated, rotate your ankles in both directions.

7. Lower Back Extension: With your feet flat on the ground and a slight forward lean, sit in a chair and reach for your toes.

8. Complete Body Stretch:- Extend your entire body by standing and extending your arms overhead.
   - To get an extra stretch, stand up on your tiptoes.

When you are stretching, always remember to breathe deeply and steadily. Instead of making any abrupt or jerky movements, you should concentrate on making soft, painless motions.


## Yoga

Yoga is an excellent and adaptable form of exercise for seniors over 50, offering a combination of physical activity, balance, flexibility, and relaxation. Here's a guide for you.

1. Warm-up:

- Begin with gentle warm-up exercises like neck rotations, shoulder rolls, and ankle circles to prepare the body.

2. Standing Poses:
  - Mountain Pose: Stand tall with feet hip-width apart, arms by the sides, and focus on steady breathing.
  - Tree Pose: Shift weight to one leg, placing the sole of the foot on the inner thigh or calf of the opposite leg.

3. Seated Poses:
  - Easy Pose (Sukhasana): Sit comfortably with crossed legs, focusing on a straight spine and relaxed shoulders.
  - Seated Forward Bend: Extend legs in front and reach towards the toes while keeping the back straight.

4. Balance Poses:
  - Warrior I and II: Step one foot back, bend the front knee, and extend arms for a gentle yet effective balance pose.
  - Modified Tree Pose: Hold onto a chair or wall for support while practicing this balance pose.

5. Floor Poses:
  - Cat-Cow Stretch: On hands and knees, alternate between arcing and rounding the back.
  - Child's Pose: Kneel and sit back on the heels, reaching arms forward for a relaxing stretch.

6. Breathing and Meditation: - Use techniques for deep breathing, like diaphragmatic or alternate nostril breathing.
   - Engage in brief guided meditation sessions or breath awareness meditation to decompress.

7. Cool Down:
   - End the session with a few minutes of relaxation in Corpse Pose (Savasana), lying on your back with eyes closed.

It's essential for you to listen to your body, avoid pushing beyond comfortable limits, and modify poses as needed. Regular yoga practice at home can contribute to improved flexibility, balance, and overall well-being for you.

## Pilates

Pilates places a strong emphasis on the body's overall conditioning, flexibility, and core strength. This is a how-to for adding Pilates to a workout regimen at home.

1. Get warmed up: To warm up the body, start with simple exercises like ankle circles, shoulder rolls, and neck tilts.

2. Mat Work:

- Pelvic Curl: While lying on your back with your knees bent, raise your hips toward the ceiling to activate your core.

- Leg Circles: While lying on your back, raise one leg and make deliberate circles in the air with it.

Marching: Make a marching motion with your legs, one at a time, while you are lying down.

3. Exercises While Seated:

- Spine Twist: While sitting with your legs outstretched, gently rotate your torso to and fro, activating your core.

Leg Stretch: Extend your legs while sitting, flex your feet, and extend your reach forward to touch your toes.

4. Exercises Done Standing:

- Heel Raises: Using your calf muscles, raise your heels off the ground while keeping your feet hip-width apart.

- Toe Taps: While standing, tap one foot forward in succession.

5. Resistance Band Work: - Use resistance bands to up the difficulty of exercises like seated rows, arm circles, and leg lifts.

6. Breathing Focus: - Engage in Pilates breathing techniques by taking a deep breath through your nose, expanding your rib cage, and fully exhaling through pursed lips.

7. Cool Down: - Conclude with mild stretches, such as the Child's Pose for relaxation or the Cat-Cow stretch from hands and knees.

 Go at your own speed, putting special emphasis on deliberate and controlled movements. Maintaining correct form is essential, and exercises should be adjusted as necessary to accommodate each person's abilities and comfort level.Seniors who regularly practice Pilates at home can benefit from increased flexibility, core strength, and general physical well-being.

# Balance and Stability Exercise:

## Tai Chi exercise

Tai Chi is a gentle and low-impact exercise that can be highly beneficial, promoting balance, flexibility, and overall well-being. Practicing Tai Chi at home provides a convenient and accessible way for seniors to reap these benefits.
Begin with a comfortable warm-up, incorporating gentle movements like arm circles and weight shifts to prepare the body for Tai Chi. These Tai Chi routines are suitable for you, making it easy to follow along at home.
Focus on the fundamental Tai Chi principles, including slow, flowing movements, controlled breathing, and mindfulness. You can start with

basic poses such as the "Ward Off" and "Grasp the Sparrow's Tail." These movements enhance balance and coordination while being gentle on joints.

As you  become more familiar with Tai Chi, you can progress to longer and more complex routines. The practice encourages joint flexibility and stability, crucial for maintaining mobility and preventing falls. Regular Tai Chi practice has been associated with various health benefits, including improved cardiovascular health, reduced stress, and enhanced mental well-being. You  should aim for at least 20-30 minutes of Tai Chi, 2-3 times per week, adjusting the duration based on your comfort and fitness level.

## Heel-to-toe walking

This is a great exercise as it improves balance and coordination. Find a clear path at home, take slow steps, placing the heel of one foot directly in front of the toes of the other. Use a support if needed, and repeat for several steps. It enhances stability and reduces the risk of falls.

## Balance exercises using a chair for support.

Chair-supported balancing exercises are beneficial. Try these out:

1. One-Leg Stands: - Cling to the rear of a robust chair.

- Raise one leg off the ground and maintain the pose for a short while.
- Change legs and repeat, lengthening the exercise gradually.

2. This is  called the heel-to-toe stand. Put one foot in front of the other so that they contact.
- For support, cling to the chair.
- Hold this stance for 20 to 30 seconds, then change your foot positioning.

3. Side Leg Raises:
   - Stand next to the chair, holding onto it for balance.
   - Lift one leg sideways and hold for a moment.
   - Lower the leg and repeat on the other side.

4. Marching in Place:
   - Lift your knees towards your chest in a marching motion while holding onto the chair for support.
   - Aim for 1-2 minutes of continuous marching.

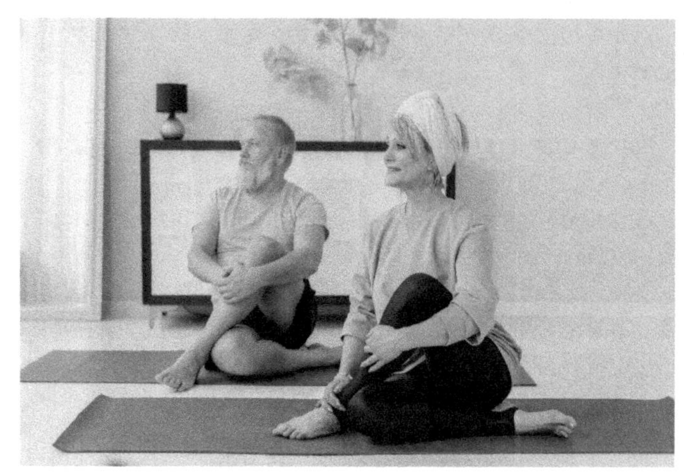

# CHAPTER FOUR

## Strength Training

1.Bodyweight Squats: - Place your feet
shoulder-width apart as you stand.
- Keep your knees in line with your toes as you slowly
descend into a squat.
Get back up while using your leg muscles.

2. Lunges: - Step forward on one foot and bend both
knees at that point in your body.
Raise yourself back up and switch to the other leg.

3. Wall Push-Ups: – Place yourself arm's length away
from a wall.
- Place your hands shoulder-height on the wall.
Keep your elbows bent and press your chest up
against the wall.

4. Chair Dips: - Take a seat on the edge of a strong
chair and hold onto it with your hands.
- Lower your body by sliding your hips off the chair,
then push yourself back up.

5. Leg Raises: - Extend one leg straight out while
seated, then hold the position for a short while.
  - Lower the leg, then switch to the opposite side.

6. Seated Marching: - Raise one leg to your chest
while sitting up in a chair.
  - Lower it, then switch to the other leg to repeat.

Always prioritize proper form over the number of repetitions. Start with a few repetitions and gradually increase as strength improves.

## Resistance band workouts

You will benefit greatly from resistance band exercises since they offer a secure and efficient means of increasing muscle mass. Here are some activities to attempt:

1. Banded Leg Press: -take a seat in a chair and wrap both legs in resistance bands, slightly above the knees.
- To overcome the band's resistance, push your knees outward.

2. Bicep Curls: - Place one or both feet in the center of the band.
- Do bicep curls while holding the band's ends with your palms facing forward.

3. Seated Rows: - Extend your legs while sitting on the floor, wrap the band around your feet, and grasp the ends.
- Grasp the band in the direction of your waist, using your upper back muscles.

4. Chest Press: - Place the band at the height of your chest.
- Using your chest muscles, hold the ends and press forward.

5. Lateral Leg Raises: - Place the band firmly on a level area.
- Lift your leg sideways against resistance and secure the other end around your ankle.

6. Tricep Extensions: - Raise both hands to grasp one end of the band.
- Raise your arms and contract your triceps.

Don't forget to select a resistance band with the right amount of tension. As strength grows, start with less resistance and progressively increase.

## light dumbbell exercise

Seated Shoulder Press:
 1. Position yourself with your feet flat on the floor and your back straight in a solid chair. With your elbows bent 90 degrees and your palms facing front, hold a light dumbbell in each hand.
When you press the dumbbells overhead, fully stretch your arms. Controllably lower them back to the beginning position. This exercise increases arm mobility and strengthens the shoulders.

Bicep Curls:
 2. Setup: Take a seat or stand with both hands holding a dumbbell, arms outstretched, and palms facing front.
As you curl the weights toward your shoulders with a biceps contraction, keep your upper arms immobile. Slowly lower the dumbbells back down.

This workout works the biceps, which are important for daily tasks.

Raises Laterally
3. Setup: Take a seat or stand with your arms at your sides, your palms facing your body, and a dumbbell in each hand.
Raise both arms to shoulder height by extending them out to the sides. Slowly lower the dumbbells back down. Better posture is encouraged by this exercise, which improves the shoulder muscles.

Advice: - Start with a weight that you can easily accomplish ten to fifteen repetitions with; - Pay attention to deliberate motions to prevent joint strain.
For seniors over 50, these exercises assist in increasing strength, flexibility, and general mobility by focusing on specific muscle groups.

## Low-Impact Aerobic Exercise

1. March in Place: - Gently raise your knees to imitate a marching gait.
   This raises your heart rate and increases muscular warmth.

2. Chair Squats: - Take a position facing a stable chair.
   Maintaining your weight on your heels, take a seat back and then stand up.

- Promotes cardiovascular health and helps build stronger leg muscles.
3. Low-Impact Jumping Jacks: Raise your arms and take one foot out to the side at a time in place of jumping.

Increases heart rate without putting joints under strain.
4. Side Leg Lifts: Use a chair as a balance aid.
   - Raise one leg and then bring it back down.
   - Fortifies thighs and hips.

5. Arm-Reach Standing March: - Raise your knee and extend the arm of the person on the other side above your head.
   - Improves balance and uses the core muscles.

6. Seated Leg March: - Place your feet flat on the ground while sitting in a chair.
   Raise one leg in a marching motion at a time.
   - Works leg muscles and improves circulation.

Crucial Advice: - Increase intensity gradually after starting off slowly.
- Aim for 150 minutes or more a week of moderate-to-intense aerobic exercise.
. Pay attention to your body and adjust the workouts to your comfort level.
Seniors over 50 can benefit from this program since it minimizes joint impact and offers cardiovascular advantages.

# Brisk walking

Although brisk walking is usually done outside, you can use a treadmill indoors or simply stroll around your house to achieve the same effect. Here's a short manual for seniors who are above 50:

1. Warm-Up: To begin, gently walk for a few minutes to loosen up your muscles.
- Gently swing your arms to improve blood flow.

2. Brisk Walking: - Keep your shoulders relaxed and your posture straight.
- Walk at a speed that increases your heart rate while still making it comfortable for you to converse.

3. Take a Walk or Use a Treadmill Indoors: - Choose a comfortable speed on a treadmill.
- Make a round around your house if you choose to stroll inside.

4. Length: - Start with at least 20 to 30 minutes.
- As your fitness level rises, gradually extend the time.

5. Cool Down: During the final few minutes, go at a slower speed to let yourself relax.
   - Stretch your quadriceps, hamstrings, and calf muscles gently.

Advice: - Put on supportive, comfy shoes.
Select a clean, well-lit space for your indoor stroll.
- Remain hydrated both before and after your stroll.

- Pay attention to the inclination and speed settings when using a treadmill.
For seniors over 50, brisk walking is a great low-impact workout that develops muscles, improves cardiovascular health, and improves general well being.

## Cycling

Cycling indoors is a great low-impact exercise for seniors
1. Stationary Bike Setup:
 - Place a stationary bike in a well-ventilated and comfortable space.
   - Adjust the seat height to ensure a slight bend in your knee when the pedal is at the lowest point.

2. Warm-Up:
   - Begin with a gentle warm-up by pedaling at a relaxed pace for 5-10 minutes.

3. Cycling Routine:
   - Cycle at a moderate pace, focusing on smooth, controlled movements.
   - Gradually increase the intensity by adjusting the resistance if your stationary bike allows.

4. Variations:
   - Incorporate intervals by alternating between periods of increased and decreased intensity.
   - Experiment with pedaling in reverse to engage different leg muscles.

5. Duration:

- Aim for 20-30 minutes initially, and gradually extend the duration as your fitness improves.

6. Cool Down:

- Finish with a cooldown period, pedaling at a slower pace for 5-10 minutes.

- Stretch your leg muscles gently after your cycling session.

Tips:

-Take note of your posture to avoid strain. Maintain a straight back, relaxed shoulders, and a small bend in your elbows.

- Use a comfortable seat cushion if needed.

- Stay hydrated during your workout.

Indoor cycling provides a cardiovascular workout, strengthens leg muscles, and is gentle on the joints, making it an excellent option for seniors.

## Seated Exercise

1. Take a comfortable seat: - Place your feet flat on the ground and your back straight when seated in a firm chair.

2. Posture: - Make sure your shoulders are relaxed and your core muscles are active.

3. Lift one leg: With one leg extended, lift it straight out in front of you.

4. Hold for a short while: - Keep your legs raised for a limited period of time while using your thigh muscles.

5. Lower leg: - Return your leg to the beginning position slowly.

6. Switch legs: - Carry out the same action on the other leg.

7. reps: - Start with 10 to 15 reps each leg, and increase as soon as it becomes comfortable.

8. Breathing: - Throughout the exercise, breathe steadily, letting out air as you raise your leg and drawing air in as you lower it.

 Benefits:
- Strengthens the muscles in your thighs.
- Improves hip flexibility.
- Enhances balance and stability.
Tips:
- Start with a height that is comfortable for lifting your leg.
- Hold onto the sides of the chair for added stability if needed.
- If you have any existing health concerns, consult with a healthcare professional before starting this or any exercise routine.
Seated leg lifts are a simple yet effective exercise for seniors, promoting strength and flexibility in the

lower body while providing a seated and stable position.

## seated marches

1. Take a comfortable seat: - Place your feet flat on the ground and your back straight when seated in a sturdy chair.

2. Posture: - Engage your core muscles and let your shoulders drop.

3. Lift one knee: Keeping the other foot on the ground, raise one knee in a marching motion towards your chest.

4. Switch legs: - Return the raised leg to its original position and raise the other knee in the same way.

5. Arm movement: Swing your arms in a natural marching beat to coordinate your actions.

6. Pace: - Move at a comfortable tempo at first, then pick up the pace if you can.

7. Repetition: - Start each leg with ten to fifteen marches, modifying as necessary.

8. Breathing:
   - Breathe steadily throughout the exercise, exhaling as you lift your knee and inhaling as you lower it.

Benefits:
- Improves circulation and warms up the body.
- Strengthens the muscles in the legs.
- Enhances coordination and balance.
Tips:
- If needed, hold onto the sides of the chair for added stability.
- Focus on controlled movements to avoid strain. Seated marches are a gentle yet effective exercise for seniors, providing a seated option that promotes leg strength, flexibility, and overall mobility.

## Water-Based Exercises

1. Water Walking: - While walking forward and backward in a shallow pool, use your core.
    - For more intensity, raise your knees.

2. Leg Lifts: - To provide support, lean on the edge of the pool.
    Elevate one leg to the front, back, and side at a time.

3. Arm Circles: - Take a stand in water up to your chest.
    - To work your shoulders, extend your arms to the sides and move them in circles.

4. Water Marching: - Move purposefully while marching in place.

- Use the water's resistance to make your muscles work.

5. Knee Lifts: - While standing in the water, raise your knees to your chest.
    - Include arm motions to work your entire body.

6. Sideways Jumps: - Leap into the water sideways and land gently.
    - Both leg strength and cardiovascular fitness are enhanced by this.

7. Exercises with Pool Noodles: - Use a pool noodle to do floating exercises, bicycle kicks, or leg kicks.
    - Increases muscle strength and flexibility in many areas of the body.

8. Torso Twists: Assume a hip-width stance and rotate your torso back and forth.
    Use your core to maintain stability.

9. Deep Water Jogging: - Jog stationary in deeper water.
    - For a more difficult workout, raise your knees and swing your arms.

10. Floating Relaxation: To unwind and stretch, spend a few minutes floating on your back.
    - Savor the water's buoyancy.

Advice: - Make sure the water is at a comfortable temperature.
- Be mindful of your body and adjust exercises as necessary.
- If you need help, use the pool stairs or something sturdy.
- Don't forget to hydrate even while in the water. Water aerobics at home provides a low-impact, effective, and enjoyable workout for seniors, promoting cardiovascular health, muscle strength, and flexibility. Always consult with a healthcare professional before starting a new exercise routine.

## Swimming

1. Stationary Swimming: -
In a smaller pool or swim spa, swim in place by alternating between flutter kicks and arm movements.
- Utilize a swim tether or resistance bands for added resistance.

3. Water Aerobics Moves:
- Incorporate traditional water aerobics exercises like leg lifts, arm circles, and knee lifts while in the water.
- Use the resistance of the water to enhance the workout.

4. Floating Exercises: - Hold onto the pool edge and float on your back.

- Perform gentle leg kicks or arm movements to engage muscles.

5. Lap Swimming: -
 If you have a longer pool, swim laps using a stroke of your choice (freestyle, breaststroke, backstroke).
- Start with a few laps and gradually increase distance.

6. Water Treading: To keep afloat, tread water vertically while utilizing your arms and legs.
   - This works a variety of muscle groups.

7. Deep Water workouts: Try deep water workouts like bicycle kicks and scissor kicks if you feel comfortable doing so.
   This increases variation and works various muscle groups.

8. Interval Training: - Mix together quick bursts of intense swimming with rest or slower swimming intervals.

   Promotes improved cardiovascular health.
Advice: - Make sure the pool is at a suitable temperature.
- Increase the length of the sessions progressively after starting with shorter ones.
- Be mindful of your body and take breaks when necessary.
- Drink plenty of water prior to, during, and after swimming.

Swimming is a full-body, low-impact exercise that offers cardiovascular benefits, muscle toning, and flexibility improvement for seniors over 50.

## Aqua jogging

1. Shallow Water Jogging: - In a swim spa or pool, stand in water that is chest deep.
   - Lift your legs and swing your arms to simulate jogging.

2. Proper Posture: - Keep your shoulders relaxed and your torso upright.
   Use your abdominal muscles to maintain stability.

3. Forward and Sideways Movement: To activate different muscle areas, jog forward and then sideways.
   - Pay attention to deliberate motions to optimize advantages.
4.High Knees: Raise your knees to a more intense sprinting position. This activates your core and works your leg muscles.

5. Arm Movement: - Swing your arms in a natural counterbalance to your legs. This makes the activity more full-body.

6. Interval Training: - Switch between sprinting at a quicker and slower pace.

- Increases calorie burning and cardiovascular fitness.

7. Treading Water:
   - Incorporate periods of water treading for added resistance.
   - Lift your knees or perform gentle kicks.

8. Incorporate Pool Accessories:
   - Use water resistance tools like aqua dumbbells or noodles to add variety to your workout.
   - Perform arm exercises while jogging.

Tips:
- Begin with a warm-up by walking in the water for a few minutes.
- Pay attention to your surroundings, especially if you're jogging in a smaller pool.
- Adjust the intensity based on your fitness level. Aqua jogging is a joint-friendly, low-impact exercise that provides cardiovascular benefits, improves muscle strength, and offers a refreshing way for seniors over 50 to stay active at home.

# CHAPTER FIVE

## Mind-Body Exercise

1. Comfortable Seating: Sit in a comfortable chair with your feet flat on the floor and hands resting on your lap.

2. Deep Breathing: Close your eyes and take slow, deep breaths. Inhale through your nose, filling your lungs, and exhale through your mouth. Focus on the sensation of each breath.

3. Body Scan: Gradually shift your attention from your breath to different parts of your body. Notice any tension or discomfort and consciously relax those areas.

4. Mindfulness of Thoughts:Allow thoughts to come and go without judgment. If your mind wanders, gently bring your focus back to your breath or the present moment.

5. Guided Imagery: Visualize a peaceful place or recall a happy memory. Engage your senses in this mental imagery.

6. Gratitude Exercise: List the things you have to be thankful for. It could be anything as basic as the comfort of sunlight or the presence of close friends and family.

7. Closing Reflection: Return your focus to the present moment gradually. Breathe deeply a few times, move your fingers and toes, and then open your eyes.

As you get more comfortable, start with shorter sessions and progressively extend them. Seniors who meditate can benefit from increased mental clarity, less stress, and overall well-being.

## Deep breathing exercise

Deep breathing exercises can be beneficial for seniors over 50. Here's a simple deep breathing routine for home:
1. Comfortable Seating: Sit in a relaxed position on a chair or cushion with your back straight and shoulders relaxed.

2. Inhalation (4 counts): Inhale slowly and deeply through your nose, counting to four. Feel your chest and abdomen expand.

3. Hold Breath (2 counts): Pause for a moment, holding the breath gently.

4. Exhalation (6 counts): Exhale slowly and completely through your mouth or nose, counting to six. Empty your lungs fully.

5. Repeat: Continue this pattern for several breath cycles. Focus on the rhythm of your breath and the sensation of air moving in and out.

6. Awareness: Pay attention to how your body feels with each breath. Notice the rise and fall of your chest and the sensation of the breath filling and leaving your body.

7. Relaxation: Release tension with each breath out. Let your face, neck, and shoulder muscles relax.

This deep breathing exercise can help seniors manage stress, improve lung capacity, and promote a sense of calm. Practice regularly, and adapt the counts based on your comfort and lung capacity.

## Mindfulness

Here's a simple mindfulness exercise for home:

1. Set a Comfortable Space: Find a quiet and comfortable place to sit or lie down. Eliminate distractions.

2. Body Scan: Close your eyes and bring attention to different parts of your body, starting from your

toes and moving up to your head. Notice any sensations without judgment.

3.Pay attention to your breathing. Sense the breath coming in and going out naturally. Refocus your thoughts softly on your breathing whenever they stray.

4. Observing Thoughts: Allow thoughts to come and go without attachment. Imagine them as passing clouds in the sky. Return your focus to the present moment.

5. Sensory Awareness: Engage your senses. Notice the sounds, smells, and sensations around you without getting caught up in them.

6. Gratitude Reflection: Take a moment to appreciate something in your life. It could be a person, a moment, or something you're thankful for.

7. Mindful Movements: Incorporate gentle movements, like stretching or reaching, with full awareness of each motion and sensation.

8. Closing Reflection: Gradually bring your attention back to the present moment. Notice how you feel and carry this sense of mindfulness into your daily activities.

Consistent mindfulness practice can enhance overall well-being, reduce stress, and improve focus. Tailor these exercises to individual comfort levels.

# Functional Movements:

## Standing from a chair

By performing this easy chair-standing exercise, seniors can increase their strength and mobility:

1. Sit-to-Stand Exercise: - Place your feet hip-width apart on the floor while sitting in a supportive chair.
   - For support, rest your hands at the edges of the chair or on your thighs.
   - Slightly bend forward and contract your abdominal muscles.
   - To stand up, drive through your heels and straighten your knees and hips.
   - Before standing, fully extend your hips.
   - Return to the chair gradually, bringing your hips up front.
Repeat: – Start with ten repetitions.

Increase the number progressively as your strength increases.

Check that the chair is steady and won't slide for safety advice.

- If necessary, add cushions or choose a higher seat.
- If needed, complete the exercise in close proximity to a stable surface for support.
- Keep a steady pace to prevent fatigue.

This workout strengthens and stabilizes the muscles in the lower body.

## Reaching exercise

Seniors over 50 can improve their flexibility and mobility with this at-home fitness routine:

1. Shoulder Reach: - Easily sit or stand.

Spread one arm out straight in front of you.

- Extend your fingers as far forward as you can while reaching.

Hold it for a short while.

- Continue with the opposite arm.

Step 2: High Reach: Place your feet hip-width apart.

Reach both arms upward and toward the ceiling.

- Extend your spine by stretching upward.

After a brief period of holding, drop your arms.

3. Side Reach: - Keep your back straight while sitting or standing.

- Lean slightly to the other side while extending one arm overhead.

- Sensate the strain on your side of the body.

Hold, then turn to face the opposite direction.

4. Diagonal Reach: - Place your feet shoulder-width apart while sitting or standing.
   - Extend one arm diagonally across your body.
   - Notice how your lower back and side are stretched.
   Hold, then go to the opposite side.

5. Toe Touches (Sitting or Standing): - Maintain a straight posture with your legs.
   - Maintain a straight back while reaching toward your toes.
   - Sensate the strain in your lower back and hamstrings.
   Hold for a little moment before stepping back into the initial position.

Don't overextend yourself; instead, always move inside your comfort zone. Regularly incorporate these reaching exercises to enhance range of motion and preserve flexibility.

## Picking Up Objects from the Floor

Improve functional strength and flexibility with this safe and effective exercise for seniors over 50:
1. Stand near a Stable Surface:
   - Position yourself close to a sturdy chair or countertop for support.

2. Feet Placement:
   - Stand with your feet shoulder-width apart.

3. Bend at the Hips and Knees:
   - Keep your back straight and bend at the hips
and knees to lower yourself.

4. Keep Objects Close:
   - If picking up a lightweight object, keep it close to
your body to reduce strain.

5. Use Proper Form:
   - Maintain a neutral spine and engage your core
as you reach down.

6. Lift with Your Legs:
   - Use your leg muscles to lift yourself back up,
rather than relying solely on your back.

7. Controlled Movement:
   - Perform the movement slowly and with control
to avoid sudden or jerky motions.

8. Repeat:
   - Start with a small object and gradually progress
to heavier items.
   - Aim for 5-10 repetitions, adjusting based on
your comfort and fitness level.

Always prioritize safety, and if needed, have
someone nearby for assistance. If you have

concerns about your ability to perform this exercise consult your doctor.

## 5 days exercise plan

This is a well-rounded, at-home 5-day fitness program for seniors over 50. Never forget to get medical advice before beginning a new workout regimen.

Day 1: Exercise with Strength
1. Sit-to-stand workouts: three sets of ten repetitions
2. Wall Push-Ups: Perform two sets of eight to ten repetitions
3. Bodyweight Squats: Three sets of eight to ten repetitions

Day 2: Cardiovascular Work
1. 15-20 minutes of brisk walking in place.
2. Marching while seated: ten minutes.
3. Ten minutes spent dancing to music.

Day 3: Balance and Flexibility
Chair yoga for fifteen minutes.
2. Leg Raises: Do two sets of ten repetitions per leg while seated.
3. Balance exercises (10 minutes) (such as standing on one leg while supported by a chair).

Day 4: Strength Training

1. Russian twists while seated: two sets of ten twists on each side.
2. Three sets of ten contractions of the abdomen while seated.
3. Plank: two sets of 15–30 seconds, if it's comfortable.

Day 5: Unwinding and Being Aware
1. Practice deep breathing for ten minutes.
2. Ten minutes of mindful walking (slow, purposeful steps).
3. 15 minutes of guided relaxation or meditation.

Never forget to stretch gently to cool down after a practice and to warm up beforehand. Pay attention to your body and adjust the exercises accordingly. Increase the duration and intensity gradually over time. For long-term advantages, consistency is essential.

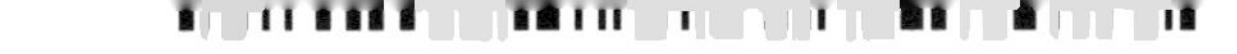

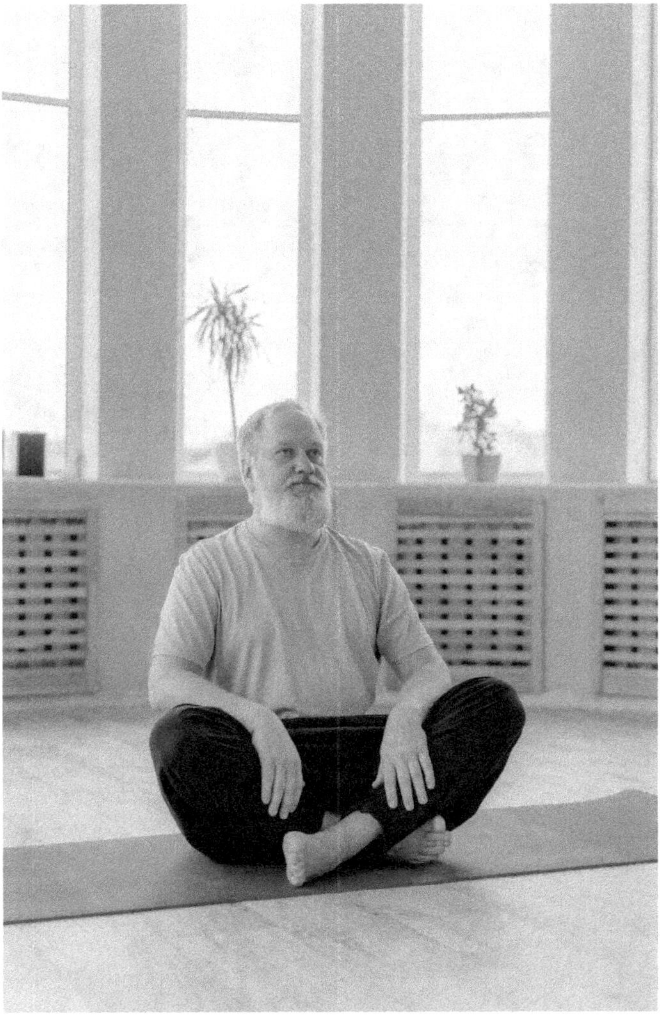

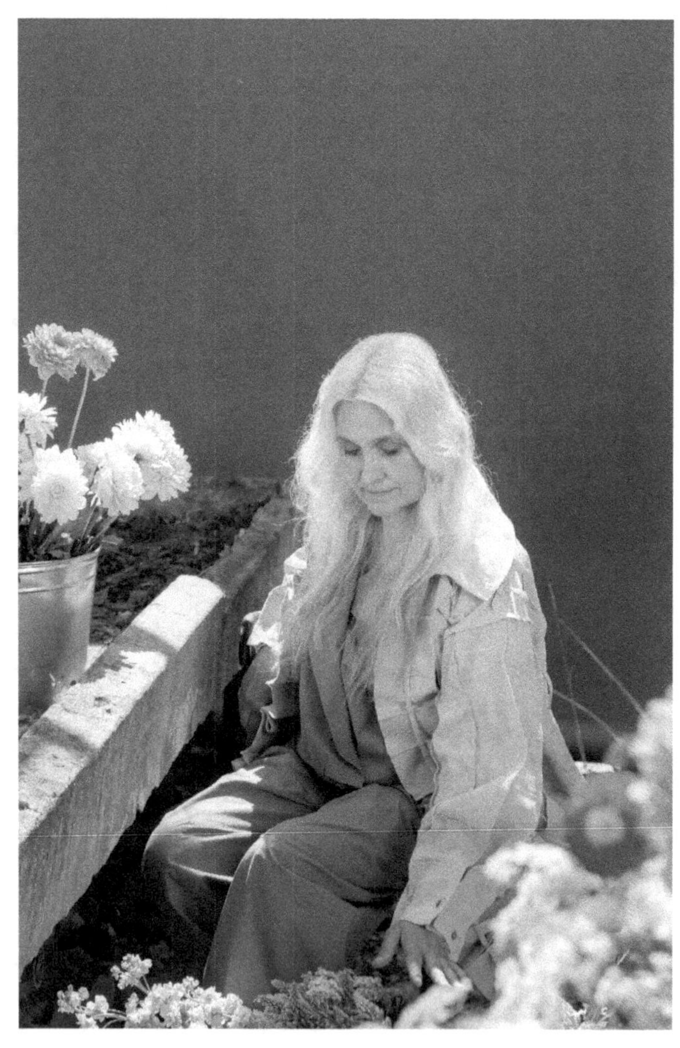

# Conclusion

Crafting a tailored home exercise routine for seniors over 50 is a key investment in health and well-being. Combining strength training, cardiovascular activities, flexibility exercises, and mindfulness creates a holistic approach to aging gracefully. Safety is paramount; hence, consultation with healthcare professionals ensures exercises align with individual health conditions. The regimen should include a mix of activities such as sit-to-stand exercises, gentle yoga or chair yoga, and cardiovascular movements like brisk walking in place. Prioritizing consistency over intensity allows gradual progress and reduces the risk of injury.

In addition to physical benefits, incorporating mindfulness and relaxation exercises contributes to mental and emotional health. Deep breathing, meditation, and mindful movements foster a sense of calm and aid in stress reduction. This comprehensive approach not only promotes longevity but also enhances the quality of life for seniors. Regular reassessment and adjustment of the exercise plan based on individual needs and capabilities are vital. Embracing a home exercise routine empowers seniors to maintain independence, improve mobility, and relish an active, fulfilling lifestyle as they navigate the golden years.

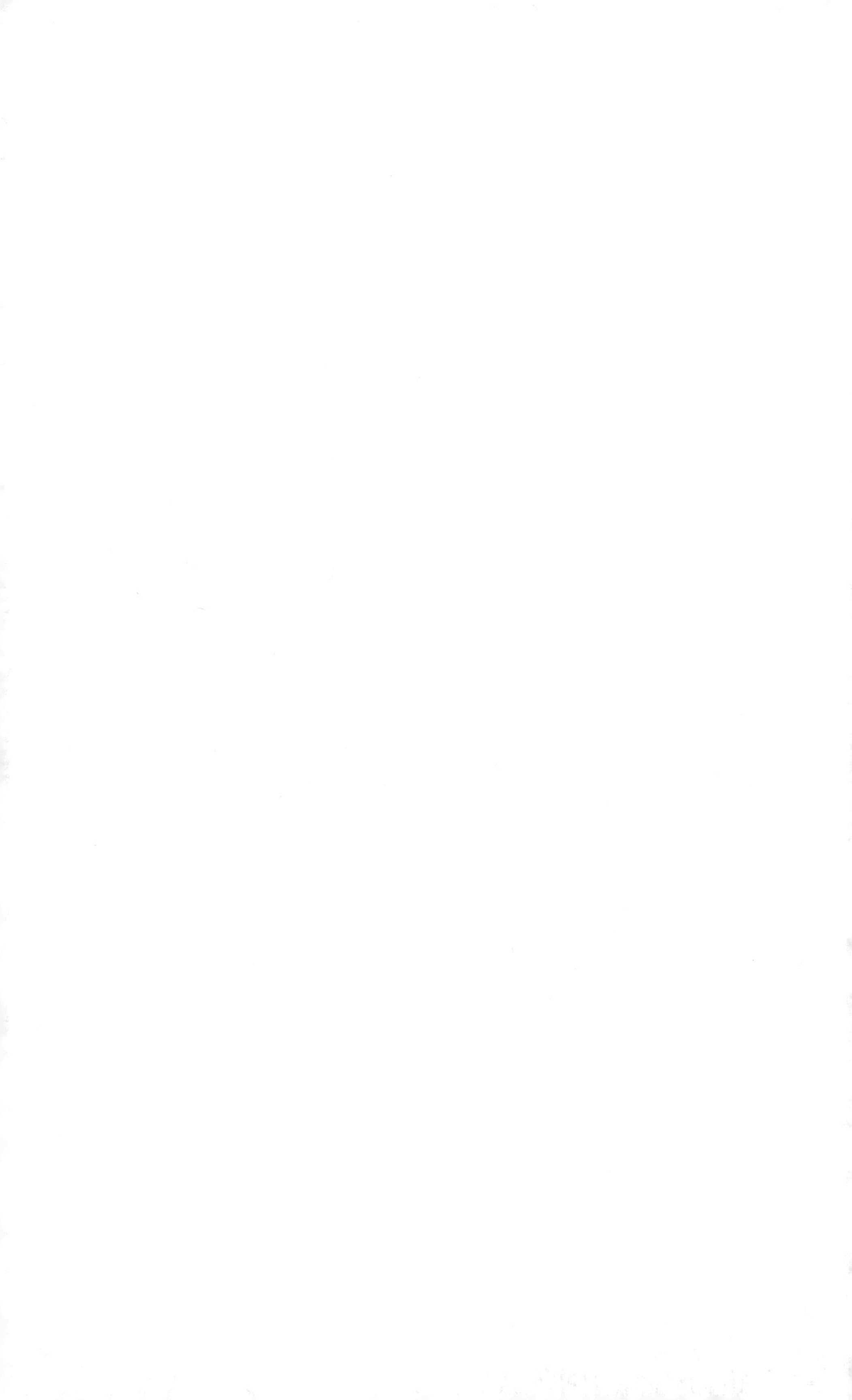